THE Holistic Lawyer

"Ritu provides practical tips on how overworked and overstressed lawyers can reconnect with themselves, their passions, and the peace that they have been missing in their lives. This book is a much-needed resource to help lawyers overcome the burnout that is all too common in our profession."

— **Ally Lozano**, Esq., Legal Business Consultant
Author of *Be the CEO of Your Law Firm*

"This book has a truly genuine and practical approach to connecting your mind, heart, and body. Ritu does a great step-by-step job at helping you become whole. *The Holistic Lawyer* is very timely in light of current health trends in the legal profession and it is bound to help many attorneys who need this support right now."

— **Fernando Flores**, Esq., High Performance Coach
and Berkeley Law Lecturer, Author of
The Essential Guide to Passing the California Bar

"With hope and clarity, Ritu shares not only the secrets of being a happier lawyer, but also the practical steps to integrate your head, heart, and spirit to create a sustainable and, dare I say it, profitable law practice. I especially appreciated the chapter on emotional intelligence, an essential skill for good lawyering."

– **Dina Eisenberg**, Esq. CEO, OutsourceEasier.com
Author of *Fiverr: The Essential Buying Guide*

"Ritu knows the intense struggles lawyers face and consequently why they burn out. She also intimately knows and lays out the holistic path for her peers to bring balance back into their lives. And she practices what she preaches. *The Holistic Lawyer* is a concise and practical guide for lawyers who are aware they need more balance and are open to wrestling with the laws of human nature, especially the law of self-sabotage."

– **Mary Ellen Hannon**, Certified Holistic Health Coach
Author of *Complementary Alternative Medicine*

"Simple, straightforward, and written from the heart, *The Holistic Lawyer* lays out a recipe for wellness and productivity accessible to all lawyers who desire balance in our practice and in our lives. Whether you are thinking about leaving the law or simply seeking to restore connection with yourself, these easy to follow steps will certainly provide clarity and the ability to see the whole picture, beginning within and permeating without."

– **Lori Bessler**, Esq., Litigator and Restorative Yoga Teacher

"This book teaches attorneys how to work with their whole brain by following six easy steps. As attorneys we are overworked all the time. There is this belief that the more hours that you work and run yourself ragged, the better an attorney you are. Some of us even brag about it. This book teaches you how to work more efficiently, more competently, and more ethically, while increasing your work-life balance."

– **Norma Lorenzo**, Esq., Hermanni & Lorenzo Law Group

"*The Holistic Lawyer* by Ritu Goswamy should be required reading for every first-year law student. It is my hope that law students could learn that in order to excel as attorneys, they need practical strategies to help them reset before experiencing work-related overwhelm. By including assignments for the reader to implement, *The Holistic Lawyer* helps law students and lawyers build a foundation of techniques to use throughout their careers. Because I have known too many lawyers who feel stuck in their legal careers, it is refreshing to read a book that uncovers the veil of dissatisfaction by offering tools to help restore a lawyer's soul."

– **Sandra Foreman**, JD, LLM, Founder, The Spa in Me, LLC

"I am (or was) the epitome of overworking to take care of clients and not taking care of myself. This book takes a deep look into the how and why we attorneys take care of others, but at the detriment to ourselves. Stop, take notice of what is truly the meaning of what we do as lawyers, and learn how to take care of yourself on such a fundamental level. This is the key to a much more balanced and happy life and law practice. Ritu has taught me how to take care of my practice by taking care of me. I am forever grateful!"

— **Shannon Englert**, Esq.

"I like to keep things really simple. The concepts that Ritu Goswamy dives into in her new book *The Holistic Lawyer* are simple. Simple, yet life changing. It's kind of like sliced bread. The technology is simple but the implementation of it can make life a whole lot easier. Learning to integrate your heart, mind, breath, and body is the foundation of what it means to be a competent lawyer. Ritu urges us to weave together these skills to step into ease and equanimity so that one's career is in concert with one's life. It's a little book with a wallop of a punch that invites the reader to open one's heart, mind, and body to serve oneself and then others—as a good lawyer should."

— **Erendira Castillo**, Esq.

THE
Holistic
Lawyer

Use Your Whole Brain to
Work Smarter Not Harder

Ritu Goswamy, Esq.

NEW YORK

LONDON • NASHVILLE • MELBOURNE • VANCOUVER

THE Holistic Lawyer
Use Your Whole Brain to Work Smarter Not Harder

© 2020 Ritu Goswamy, Esq.

Published in New York, New York, by Morgan James Publishing in partnership with Difference Press. Morgan James is a trademark of Morgan James, LLC. www.MorganJamesPublishing.com

ISBN 978-1-64279-619-3 paperback
ISBN 978-1-64279-620-9 eBook
Library of Congress Control Number: 2019938317

Cover Design by:
Rachel Lopez
www.r2cdesign.com

Interior Design by:
Bonnie Bushman
The Whole Caboodle Graphic Design

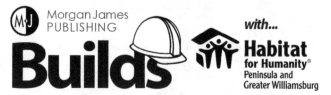

Morgan James is a proud partner of Habitat for Humanity Peninsula and Greater Williamsburg. Partners in building since 2006.

Get involved today! Visit
www.MorganJamesBuilds.com

To Angie Boissevain, poet and Zen teacher,
for teaching me the power of being silent.

In memory of Ken Kezeor, my neighbor and
friend, who built supports for me during
the writing of this book.

Table of Contents

Foreword

The core elements of transforming your life are healing your past and empowering your future. As a transformational psychologist and a chiropractor I have studied the neurology and unique processes that result in lasting personal development. I have experienced first-hand how having an integrated whole brain gives you access to and encourages the advanced development of your forebrain, which is the CEO of your life. I currently work as a business consultant with influential leaders who are ready to take their life and work up to the next level—creating transformation for their clients and the world.

I have come to know Ritu Goswamy first as a fellow author and then as my client. Ritu is truly an influential leader with her work with lawyers and it is a pleasure to watch her step into her power with this role. Ritu has been on her own journey to learn how lawyers, such as herself, can have a bigger impact and relieve conflict in the world without burning themselves out. While she is certainly qualified to do the work she does with lawyers, it's impressive to watch how she continues to grow and learn as she teaches others.

Her first book for lawyers, *The New Billable Hour*, was wonderful guidance for incorporating simple lifestyle practices for increased productivity. This book, *The Holistic Lawyer*, takes the lawyer to the next level. Using the whole brain perspective, Ritu takes the lawyer through a six-step process of reintegrating the brain. Not only does she accessibly explain basic neuroscience, she teaches practical exercises lawyers specifically can easily implement into their lives. And yes, this process will definitely result in the lawyer working smarter, not harder.

My son is a lawyer, and I have seen how he has used the law to transform those around him. When he walks into a room, he commands respect and people listen to him. He did not get here by merely aggressively working hard. He has practiced what Ritu lays out in her Holistic Lawyer formula: he connects head, heart, and gut to practice law from a centered and expansive place. Rather than creating drama and disconnection, he brings people together in creative solutions. I am deeply impressed with my son and can only imagine how the world would be a different place if we had more lawyers like him.

Thank goodness Ritu has created a system to create such lawyers! If you are a lawyer and are ready to go to the next level of your success and want to make a bigger impact in your role, this book is for you. And if you are feeling exhausted and your current model of work isn't serving you anymore, this book will help you turn things around and look at your work differently. I am confident that lawyers can be influential leaders and Ritu will show you how to get there. *The Holistic Lawyer* is an accessible, practical blueprint for lawyers who want maximum success.

—**Dr. Ron Stotts**, Transformational Business Guide
Author of *Overscheduled by Success: A Guide for Influential Leaders Too Busy to Create Their Next Dream*

Introduction
Who Is This "Holistic Lawyer"?

I first put the word "holistic" with "law" shortly after law school, before "holistic" became trendy. To me, "holistic" was just another way to say "whole"—to express that we have to be careful not to be myopic in our role as lawyers. It was clear to me that in order to be effective lawyers, we needed to see the "whole picture." The law school training at the time was to analyze a fact pattern and narrow our focus by "issue-spotting." I was perturbed by this way of problem solving. How can we resolve conflict in people's lives while essentially ignoring what was going on behind the scenes?

How could we resolve the issue at hand without stepping back and considering the problem from all angles?

My existential angst led me to pursue a joint degree after I had already begun law school. After my first year of law school, I joined the graduate school of social work in the same university and studied law and social work at the same time. In five years, I had earned both a Juris Doctorate and a Master of Social Work.

As you may know, the social work profession is very holistic. As a social worker, you are trained to constantly look at the big picture. A client or organization may come to you with one problem, which is usually a symptom of some other cause or causes. It was in social work school that I learned about systems theory and how one imbalance or change in a part of a system affects the whole thing. This made sense to me.

Then cut back to law school, where I was still engaged in the intellectual rigor. I enjoyed the challenge of finding what was "wrong" in a situation, who to blame, and how to achieve a sense of justice. I relished (and still do) the idea of being an advocate, a hero, and a leader who had the power to make a difference in the world. Being a lawyer was both prestigious and intimidating to others. It is a profession that I (and my parents) could be proud of.

On the other hand, being a social worker is not as respected. Even though the education and practical training that I received have given me a unique lens from which to practice law, I have downplayed them. I have held myself out to be a lawyer first and foremost and have had a successful career serving my law clients in a holistic way. The first half of my career—about 8 years—was in the nonprofit sector working for several legal services organizations. Then, over 10 years ago, I started my own law firm, Holistic Legal Services.

The approach of Holistic Legal Services is to treat the client as a whole person. But it also is about the lawyer bringing his or her whole self to the work with the client. The whole lawyer, or the holistic lawyer, is present, focused, sharp, compassionate, willing, understanding, assertive, strong, and ready to guide the client through a confusing and complex experience within the legal system. By providing holistic legal services, the lawyer can bring the client to a better understanding of the client's situation and also provide some perspective to ground the client as she experiences the legal system firsthand.

As I have practiced law in this way, and pursued my own healing and spiritual path, I experienced mutual alchemy with my clients. We essentially transform each other. I have a deep understanding of the healing work a lawyer does. And if you also truly want to change lives and do meaningful work as a lawyer, it starts with changing how you practice law.

By committing to become a "holistic lawyer," you are setting the intention to not only see the "whole picture" of your clients' cases, but are also striving to reconnect with lost parts of yourself that will help you work (and live) more easefully, creatively, generously, and yes, more intelligently!

The legal profession needs to upgrade and innovate to keep up with other professions and the dynamic modern world. And as lawyers, now is the time to develop new ways to hone our craft. Lawyers are not going obsolete. We are needed more than ever to heal conflict and empower our clients. It is due to this insight that I no longer hide my vision that all lawyers can be holistic. Holistic is no longer a new age phenomenon for the "soft" sciences. It is for everyone, especially lawyers.

Together we can increase our impact and success as lawyers if we embrace new ways of thinking and being. By being holistic, we are always considering the whole picture and we are continuously accessing more of ourselves. This is the holistic lawyer and the future of the legal profession.

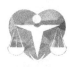

Chapter 1
The Overworked Lawyer

Work
Yet life is not a vision nor a prayer,
But stubborn work; she may not shun her task.
After the first compassion, none will spare
Her portion and her work achieved, to ask.
She pleads for respite, —she will come ere long
When, resting by the roadside, she is strong.
– Emma Lazarus

L awyers work hard. Like, really hard. And we work this hard because we know how to push our intellect to its limit and, in some cases, beyond its limit. You probably enjoy working hard and that's great. Your dedication to your work is admirable and impressive. The legal profession is based on this notion of working hard to be a competent and ethical professional. You have complied with these high standards of the field and have a successful career for it. This paradigm of working hard and pushing your limits has served you well. Achieving success by working hard has given you results and validation.

Your hard work began even before you became a lawyer. You toiled many hours in law school and in studying for the bar. However, any glamour of being a lawyer has become eclipsed by paperwork and research. Even though it is impossible to know everything, you have to try to learn as much as possible in order to be competent. The numerous ethical rules taunt you to push harder for fear of making a mistake and having a complaint filed against you. And you have come to accept that being a lawyer means sacrifice. Working is a big part of your identity. Other lawyers and non-lawyers alike have reinforced this notion that lawyers are *over*worked, *over*burdened, *over*whelmed, and *over*stressed.

I once told my legal assistant that I felt overwhelmed. She replied with a crooked smile, "Are you really? Maybe you are just pleasantly whelmed." I loved that. Why do we *over*do things? Why can't we stop working?

Given the rapid pace of changing law, it is no wonder that due diligence can lead to overworking. To show our clients and ourselves that we are truly competent, we must hit the books and keep researching until we feel confident in our legal advice and strategic decisions. But the truth is that we rarely feel confident that we have completed our research. It is impossible. Nevertheless, the clients are counting on us! We are driven by this responsibility that may sometimes feel like a burden. And on top of that, the legal culture encourages overwork.

In my first book, *The New Billable Hour*, I tackled head-on the topic of the billable hour system for lawyers and how we must change that measure of our own worth. Due to under-billing and low collection rate, the billable hours just don't add up. And our downfall as lawyers is non-billable, non-productive time spent away from living the life we deserve. We want to do a good job, but *there just aren't enough hours in the day to bill clients.*

That is why I created the New Billable Hour™ program. It's simple; you bill yourself one hour per day, every day, for increased productivity and work-life balance. This notion of billing yourself first is in line with paying yourself first, or the "profit first" model. Since lawyers' profitability is based on the billable hour, I outlined a system where you bill yourself *before* billing clients. By billing yourself first, you will bill more hours to clients.

The New Billable Hour book and system has changed the lives of many lawyers who have implemented the simple practices into their daily lives. They report being more calm, more present, more balanced, more productive, and more confident in their ability to make decisions. The lawyers who have learned the system have wanted more; they have wanted to even further upgrade their practice of law. They wanted more confidence and to know how to work smarter, not harder.

And that is why I wrote this book. *The Holistic Lawyer* is the next level after the foundational book and program of *The New Billable Hour.* This book and program will help you learn how to practice law by using your whole brain and self to truly work smarter. Just like we outgrew the archaic billable hour system, we have outgrown how we learned to use our brains and the traditional definition of being smart. That idea of being "smart" has meant that we have been overusing certain parts of our brains to our detriment. We overwork since we cannot possibly accomplish our goals in the way we have been operating. What if using your whole brain, being holistic, could mean accomplishing everything you desire?

Modern times have led to imbalances in how we work. We tend to favor some parts of ourselves and ignore others. This dismissal of parts of ourselves leaves us feeling disconnected, incomplete, and isolated. When we feel this way, we can set out to reconnect with ourselves to feel whole, complete, and integrated with the world around us.

Even as a lawyer, you can reconnect to yourself to become whole. Those parts you may have ignored or suppressed can be reawakened and reintegrated. To succeed, you had to separate out parts of yourself—and it worked! Every choice, strategy, decision, and sacrifice got you here to this moment. You made it to this exact moment. You are a successful lawyer, even if you don't always feel that way about the success part.

I know that to a lawyer, these ideas of being whole or holistic seem grand. And of course they are enormously huge ideas. Warning! These ideas could be lifechanging. I could be leading you to the end of your legal career. You probably have regular thoughts of leaving the profession for a more neutral career, like a barista. And maybe this holistic talk will put you over the edge. Wait a minute, hold on, and back away from the coffee shop. Hear me out.

The holistic lawyer is like a super lawyer. When you learn how to tap into who you really are, your legal career will be enhanced, you will have access to so many more resources than you can ever imagine, and you will have clarity in your choices. So your next steps, whether in or out of the profession, will be clear and drama-free. You won't be running anymore. You will gently glide to your next step.

In *The New Billable Hour*, I taught you about mindfulness: focusing your mind on the present moment throughout your day. This book is about connecting and integrating your mind/brain/head with the rest of your whole being. And that is why this book is called *The Holistic Lawyer*. Change is here and you are not alone. There is a better way to think, learn, and practice law. And it starts with you. Keep reading to learn how.

Chapter 2
The Whole Brain Perspective

The Brain Is Wider than the Sky
The Brain—is wider than the Sky—
For—put them side by side —
The one the other will contain
With ease—and You—beside—

The Brain is deeper than the sea—
For—hold them—Blue to Blue—
The one the other will absorb—
As Sponges—Buckets—do—
— **Emily Dickinson**

L awyers pride ourselves on being smart and using our brains. However, there is so much more of your brain that you have to discover. What we have learned about being smart is only part of the story. In our pursuit of being a good student and good lawyer, we have, unfortunately, disconnected from parts of our brains and ourselves. We are fragmented and long to be whole.

But, how *do* you reconnect with yourself to become whole? You will first need to shift your own paradigm of how your brain relates to the rest of your being. Let's start with some basic neuroscience and how the brain functions. (If you are interested in more detailed information, check out the "Further Reading" page at the end of this book.)

The brain is the commander in chief of the nervous system. And the nervous system controls all our body systems. According to science, the brain is powerful and almighty. It is therefore worth taking a closer look at the brain. The human brain has three parts, which have each evolved over time. Our oldest and most primitive part of the brain is the instinctual, or reptilian, brain. We share this primitive brain with a lot of animals. This is the part of the brain responsible for survival and the "flight or fight" response. If a tiger were chasing you, this part of the brain would release neurochemicals, including adrenaline, to help you to react quickly. The primitive brain allows you to act in an emergency. So when you need to act quickly out of fear, you can attack or run away.

Lawyers feel like we are constantly being chased. We are literally poised to fight at any given moment. And it comes from all sides. We lawyers formally fight in court as litigators. And we also fight systems and policies as advocates for our clients. Moreover, as lawyers, we are constantly fighting *potential* threats to our clients. We use this primitive part of the brain to stay in a state of constant hypervigilance. By staying in emergency mode, we are ready at any given moment to react to threats.

The old-school primitive brain has helped to keep us alert. Then, over time, evolution has created a second part of the brain: our emotional, or limbic, brain. This means, like a lot of other animals, we have the ability to have emotions. Our emotions evolved to serve the reptilian brain and warn us about danger. An emotion is a feeling that arises in us. *Emotions are energy in motion.* We develop problems when we don't let this energy move. It is important to note that our emotions mean something. And our emotions are wrapped up in memories to make them feel even more intense.

Emotional imbalance occurs when we either express too much emotion or too little.

Unfortunately, as lawyers we tend to avoid processing our emotions. Even though we have this ability to feel, we have learned that the "soft skill" of being "touchy feely" is not respectable or necessary for a lawyer. So, as a result, we either ignore our emotions or try to escape them. Conversely, we also tend to perseverate on our negative emotions, like anger or resentment, to fuel our fight. While anger does help us fight, holding on to this emotion causes us more harm than good.

Our brain detects and holds on to negative information faster than positive information. And negative experiences leave a trace in the brain, ready to reactivate if you encounter a similar event. As lawyers, we are constantly faced with negative situations. You know what they say: "You don't like lawyers until you need one." And you need one when something negative happens in your life. The lawyer is constantly hit with the negative. When clients ask me whether others are having problems in their cases, I reply that I have a bias because I only know about problems—not when things are going well. It is the nature of my job as a lawyer.

However, by actually paying attention to our emotional brain, we can better manage the stress of emergencies handled by the primitive brain. That's great news. But wait! There's more. There is yet another part of the brain for us to use. The third and newest part of our brain, which sets humans apart from many other animals, is the neocortex, or intellectual brain. While the first two parts of the brain keep us alive, this part of the brain allows us to thrive. The neocortex is divided into two hemispheres—the right and the left. The left side is the part responsible for logical, linear reasoning and the right side is the creative, spatial-visual side and handles intuition. The creative right side of the brain is enhanced with movement, art, or music. This part of the brain, the neocortex, when both sides are integrated, is where deep wisdom resides.

As lawyers, we have lost that integration of both sides of the neocortex. We tend to overuse the left side, and neglect the right side. When we overwork, we let physical activity go. We let that art interest we had before law school go. And what happens is that when you don't use it, you lose it. So the right side is not used and the left side gets overused and fatigued. When the sides are not integrated, we are not as smart. If we can use our intuition and creativity to look at the big picture, we will do a better job with the details of our work as lawyers.

Do you feel like you lost part of yourself since law school? In my first book, *The New Billable Hour*, I shared with you an example of how one lawyer stopped doing the outdoor activities he was passionate about. And from there, slowly other activities shifted to the wayside. I hear time and time again that lawyers have no life outside of work. Of course, there are many lawyers who do have creative hobbies, raise families, and nurture plants/animals/people. In fact, most lawyers have that creative outlet that they are either doing or wish they were doing. I know you have one. Or two. Whether it's surfing, dancing, cooking, painting, or mountain biking, you have a deep desire to balance the left side with these right side activities. This is the whole brain perspective.

It is important to understand that humans did not evolve to rid ourselves of the older parts of our brains, but to add layers of new on top of old. This layering is what keeps integrating what came before. Our intellectual brain helps us properly manage both our instinctual brain and emotional brain. However, when we are overworked and stressed out, we rely on only our primitive and emotional brains. And when we favor the left side of the neocortex and ignore the right side, we are also causing fatigue. In this imbalanced state, we are not managing anything. We are merely letting our brains control *us*. This was the motivation for me to write this book—are lawyers using our whole brains?

When lawyers access our whole brains, amazing insights, strategies, and decisions are continually born. I am sure you know how it feels when things click and your analysis just flows. And you also know how it feels to only use parts of your brain. You feel imbalanced, stressed, and anxious. When we are not using all the parts of our brains as a whole, we are not working as efficiently as we could be.

What if you could integrate all of who you are to feel more ease, balance, productivity, and success? What if you could have more impact and make more money too? What if you could enjoy lawyering more, and that enjoyment rippled out to your clients, opposing counsel, judges, and the entire profession? What if you could integrate the parts of your brain to actually work smarter and not harder? Sound interesting? Then this book is for you. Keep reading.

Chapter 3

The Holistic Lawyer

A Dream Within a Dream
You are not wrong, who deem
That my days have been a dream;
Yet if hope has flown away
In a night, or in a day,
In a vision, or in none,
Is it therefore the less gone?
All that we see or seem
Is but a dream within a dream.
– Edgar Allan Poe

When I learn new ways of thinking and working, it doesn't feel real. Little by little, the way I had learned to work and be a competent lawyer begins to unravel, like it was all a dream. I understand that while the concepts I will teach you are simple, they will seem strange and unreal to you. And that is okay. Through the steps you will learn how to shift your perspective to create a new way of working that will indeed allow you more access to your brain so you can work smarter.

In the following six chapters, I will teach you a process I created based on the work I have done myself and taught my lawyer clients. This holistic lawyer program is a guide to reintegrate your brain to optimal performance levels and give you the tools to stop overworking. As you know, the New Billable Hour program is your foundation and the prerequisite for this program. (I will review the steps for that program in the next chapter.)

Just like the New Billable Hour, this program is divided into six lessons and each lesson builds on the prior one. Everything you learn will build on everything that came before it. You will practice each lesson for a period of time (at least a week) and then add the next lesson, and so forth. As you will see, becoming holistic means activating your whole brain—which means that your goal is to ultimately master all the lessons simultaneously. But, initially, try each lesson and do your best to maintain it as you layer on the next lesson. Later, with help or on your own, you can go back and further practice the lessons that were difficult for you.

The Holistic Lawyer Program:

- Lesson One: Cultivate Daily Mindfulness: Beyond the New Billable Hour
- Lesson Two: Connect Mind + Body: Breathe Deeply
- Lesson Three: Connect Brain + Gut: Think with Your Belly
- Lesson Four: Connect Head + Heart: Raise Your Emotional IQ
- Lesson Five: Depose Yourself: The Self-Inquiry Process
- Lesson Six: Find Your Purpose: Your Mission Statement

In Lesson One you will learn how to cultivate daily mindfulness, going beyond the New Billable Hour. In this first lesson, you will make sure you are practicing the minimum of billing yourself one hour per day before you bill clients. The New Billable Hour is meant to be aspirational and not to be done perfectly each and every day. If you have easily added a particular lesson into your day as habit, increase the time you spend for that activity. Then, note the lessons that have been difficult for you, and focus on those "stuck" places. Develop awareness for when and why those lessons go by the wayside when you don't bill yourself first.

In Lesson Two you will learn how to connect your mind and body through your breath. This is the most important lesson that you can use in your life. This lesson is about breathing into whatever is going on around you and continuing to create awareness. So this lesson is very profound—obviously, because you are breathing deeply—and it is something that you will want to carry with you everywhere all the time. Even just incorporating one conscious breath into your day is connecting your body and mind.

In Lesson Three you will learn how to connect your brain and gut and think with your belly. In this lesson, I will guide you to practice using your intuition to develop your confidence as a lawyer. Events can be happening within you (internal chaos) or outside of you (external chaos), but by connecting to your gut, you can have a nice foundation to face the world and do your best.

As you know from the New Billable Hour Program, the first three lessons of my programs are fundamental and then the lessons become a little more challenging.

In Lesson Four you will learn how to connect your head with your heart and raise your emotional intelligence. You will identify and observe your emotions so you can become intelligent in identifying them. As I explained in the last chapter, there is immense power and possibility in connecting with your emotional brain.

In Lesson Five you will learn how to depose your*self!* This lesson takes emotional intelligence a step further through a process I call "The Self-Inquiry Process." You will learn how to use the identification and observation of emotions as signals to process thoughts, history, and ultimately what is happening in the present moment.

In Lesson Six you will learn how to create your own mission statement for your life and work. Without a mission, you are traveling an arduous road instead of journeying on a joyful path of self-discovery. By the end of the program, you will have created a destination for your career and life map, and this will make all the difference in how you choose to use your brain.

How to Use this Book:

I suggest that you first read *The New Billable Hour* to have a foundation for what you are about to learn. (In case you are not able to read it right now, or if it has been a while since you did, I provide a short summary of that book and program in the next chapter.) Then, please read this book once all the way through for context. At the end of each chapter I offer an assignment to complete over the course of at least a week. As you read the chapters and assignments the first time around, you may implement some of the ideas into your life and work.

Finally, after you get the whole picture, go back and read the lessons one at a time and take some time, at least a week, to do each assignment. Once you feel like you understand a lesson, move on to the next lesson and layer on the next assignment. Take as long as you need to stay with a lesson. My clients work this program for about a year. However, each person has her own speed and way of learning. As you move from one lesson to the next, remember to keep the prior assignments active as you add more assignments. In other words, each lesson is simply fleshing out the ones before it, including the basics of the New Billable Hour Program, to guide you on how to live a whole brain lifestyle.

The lessons are not meant to be burdens, but a way to expand your awareness of how you can more fully use your brain to work smarter. As you move through your life, you will develop the ability to draw upon which lessons are necessary to enhance your brain in that moment. Sound like a dream? Well it is. Don't overthink it. Just trust that you are about to take a journey to learn how to live the life of your dreams.

Are you ready? Grab your lawyer baggage…I mean luggage…and let's go.

Chapter 4
Lesson One:
Cultivate Daily Mindfulness:
Beyond the New Billable Hour

The Balloon of the Mind
Hands, do what you're bid:
Bring the balloon of the mind
That bellies and drags in the wind
Into its narrow shed.
– W.B. Yeats

The terms "brain" and "mind" are often used interchangeably. But what is the difference? Well, the brain is the physical organ I described in Chapter 2. And the mind, not just confined to the brain, is responsible for your thoughts, feelings, attitude, and imagination. So when we talk about using your whole *brain*, this means also harnessing the power of your *mind*.

"Mindfulness" is a practice where we take control of our wandering mind—in theory. What we are really doing is using the power of our mind to be in the present moment. One way we do this is through meditation—which is just a formalized practice of avoiding distractions and practicing being mindful in the moment. Since these concepts appear to be esoteric when you have a polluted or distracted mind, meditation for lawyers is key.

I know that sitting quietly and focusing on your breath can be challenging for the average lawyer. And that is why it is *necessary* for the holistic lawyer. By learning how to get quiet and be present, you can use your mind (and brain) instead of letting it use you. The first lesson of this program is to cultivate mindfulness in the form of regular daily meditation.

My meditation teacher once told me that our meditation practice is like a boiling pot of water. If we turn it off (miss a session), then we have to put in more energy to get the pot boiling again. But if we are consistent with our practice, we keep the pot boiling, and enjoy the constant simmer of our lives. Then we don't have start up again. This is like anything—like exercise or diet—when we stop, it takes a lot to get back into it.

In *The New Billable Hour*, I presented to you my system for billing yourself one hour per day for your mindfulness practices. The lessons in this book build upon that foundation.

Let's review the six-step New Billable Hour program:

Step 1: Meditate (.1 hour)
Step 2: Take a real lunch break (.2 hour)
Step 3: Create an energizing morning routine (.2 hour)
Step 4: Create a grounding night routine (.2 hour)
Step 5: Incorporate movement with breath (.2 hour)
Step 6: Connect with nature (.1 hour)

In implementing this system, there are three rules to consider:

Rule 1: Try your best to bill what you are supposed to bill. Set the intention and make the effort.

Rule 2: No double billing…yet. For the initial program, make sure you bill each separate activity for the time required. If you do them simultaneously, just add the required time.

Rule 3: Restart from the beginning every day. At the end of the day, go to sleep knowing you tried your best. Then you start the next day anew. You cannot make up missed hours or bill ahead.

The New Billable Hour program is an introduction to mindfulness practice. In that book, you learned how to practice mindfulness in six different ways. The mindful eating exercise of the lunch break is especially challenging for lawyers to do. Paying attention to what you are doing first thing in the morning and last thing at night was likely eye-opening for your awareness. It was not important what you actually did in those routines or if you did the same routines every day. The point of the program was to pay attention to where you were, what you did, and how you did it without distractions. The distractions are the opposite of mindfulness. Mindfulness is actually paying attention to what you are doing. This is so easy that it can be difficult because it involves letting go and really seeing how things are.

Mindfulness is paying attention to what you are doing in the present moment. It is about showing up and really listening to yourself. Now that you know how to cultivate mindfulness for one hour per day, you will want to do it for all of your hours. I know this notion is likely mind-blowing. That is the essence of mindfulness—it blows your mind. The endgame is to live our lives in that mindful state, a state that may have been uncomfortable for you. Believe me, I understand the resistance. I have to admit that I have argued with my current teacher about wanting a "break" from my mindfulness practices. He simply replies, "You want a break from being conscious?" Being conscious is what will make you smarter in the long run.

In this book, we take mindfulness to the next level. And just like the New Billable Hour lessons, there will be some lessons that will be easy for you and some that need to be revisited. It is not about doing everything perfectly, but about creating more awareness in your life about how you do things. When you start practicing mindfulness, you are watching your life and you are able to see boundaries between where you end and where other people begin. This also applies when you experience the news, legal updates, opposing counsel, and clients. If you can use your mind to integrate your whole brain, and become a holistic lawyer, you will be a better lawyer because you won't be so reactive. You will respond instead of react. With every breath, you will let life live through you and not have to push so hard. When we integrate ourselves, we show up more fully in our relationships, communicate better with our clients, excel in our work, and enhance every aspect of our lives. We can treat ourselves better since lawyers tend to beat ourselves up.

To cultivate mindfulness, you must have a daily meditation practice. The goal is not to meditate all day and night. It is not like the more you meditate, the better you do. Keep up all your New Billable Hour practices. But the sitting meditation is most important. The reason is because when we are just sitting, we can really allow our thoughts to calm down and tap into the power of the mind.

Lesson One Assignment:

At this point in your journey, schedule your meditation practice for twice a day, preferably at the same times of day. Ideally your two sessions would be first thing in the morning and then in the evening time (either before dinner or before you go to sleep). It may be difficult to stay awake in the night meditation if you are tired, so experiment with when works for you. You don't want to be too hungry, or too full, or too tired. Find a time that works for you in the morning and evening to sit quietly and comfortably in meditation. The sessions can be a minimum of .1 hours (six minutes) each and you will gradually increase the time. Since you are already meditating once a day, simply add an additional session for at least that amount of time.

If you are not doing your meditation twice per day, just notice why. Is it because you are too tired? Then change the time. Are you forgetting? Set a reminder. Whenever you implement a big change in your life, it takes discipline at first. And then when you develop this new habit, you will simply crave it. Your meditation practices will be a natural part of your life. You will forget less. It will be like anything else you do that you love. It will become part of the fabric of your life.

That being said, we are using the same rules as the New Billable Hour. Do not beat yourself up. If you are exhausted, go to sleep. If you are traveling or people are visiting you, just do your best. If you are sick or something gets in the way of your meditation, it is okay, just pick up where you left off.

Chapter 5
Lesson Two:
Connect Mind + Body:
Breathe Deeply

An ancient pond…
An ancient pond!
With a sound from the water
Of the frog as it plunges in.
– Matsuo Basho

31

A h, we all revel in the simple pleasures of life. So then why do we make life so difficult by separating body from mind? According to modern science, we used to think the mind and body were separate. That was how modern medicine operated until recently. Over time, research has shown that the body and mind are connected and one influences the other. This body-mind connection means that we can't have one without the other. For example, if you wanted to raise your hand, your mind has to communicate with your body. They are connected.

The latest research is finally confirming that the mind and body are one. They are so intimately connected that they are the same thing. In fact, we have a "body-mind." Ancient wisdom has already known that we can influence our body with our mind; modern science continues to confirm this. For example, the placebo effect has proven that we can use our minds to influence what happens to our bodies. If our bodies are ill, this affects our minds. If our bodies are not doing well, we are going to have mental health problems.

We also know that the systems of the body are working together. The circulatory system, digestive system, and all others are working together and controlled by the nervous system, which is led by the brain. So the brain is controlling all of our systems. However, somewhere along the way of becoming a lawyer, we have not kept up with science.

We still think that being in our heads and overusing our brains is the correct choice. We tend to overdo it and fatigue ourselves. As I explained in *The New Billable Hour*, we ignore how our body is responding to this overworking of the mind. We think the body and mind are separate and we may cover up the symptoms of that disconnect. This is why there are rampant substance abuse problems, mental health issues, and suicides in the legal profession. It is because we are ignoring the body-mind connection. We are not treating them as one thing. We tell ourselves that we can just push through the stress. But we can't. The day of reckoning has arrived.

It is time for you to reconnect your mind and body. And there's good news: you can do this through your breath. And that is something that you have all of the time. You don't have to pay for it. It's free! It's accessible. You would be surprised about how much we are not using this resource. With my clients and even the lawyers I do consultations with, I ask what they are doing to manage their stress. They often respond that they are doing "breathing exercises," or simply that they are breathing. In your day-to-day life, notice when you are not breathing fully. You may be breathing enough for survival, enough for flight or fight, enough to get through a situation, but not enough to be thriving.

When you constrict your body and your breathing through your mind and your thinking, your brain cannot be expansive as it could be. So think about how the objective of this book is to learn how work smarter, not harder. You are working really hard on a little bit of oxygen!

You are working in this emergency mode, when you can be more expansive. I am going to call this concept the "breath" because it is the most accessible term. But this is also called chi, energy, life force, spirit, or whatever is moving through us that you believe in. I am going to be talking about the yoga discipline, because that is my background. In yoga this concept is called "prana." If you break down this Sanskrit word, "pra" means movement and "na" means constant. So prana means constant movement.

The chapter in *The New Billable Hour* about movement and connecting it with breath is basically this. We are constantly moving and the life force is moving. The good news is that we ourselves are the ones causing any constriction in that movement. We are the ones stopping it and not letting it flow. The movement of the prana is what yoga does. Yoga is a breath practice. In practicing yoga, we are reconnecting body-mind. (In addition to yoga, other ancient practices such as qigong and tai chi are also about moving energy with breath.)

Another yogic practice is "pranayama," which translates to "breath control." When you do guided meditations with your mobile app or with a teacher, that is what you are doing—you are controlling the breath. You are helping it flow more easily. Pranayama practice does not have to be extreme. For you, holistic lawyer in training, pranayama means paying attention to your breath and breathing expansively.

As lawyers, we are often holding our breath or not breathing as much as we can be. You tend to restrict your breathing. That is what anxiety is; you aren't breathing fully. In law school, I suffered from panic attacks, and it felt like I could not breathe. When I felt an attack coming on, I would go back to my apartment, get in bed, and pull the covers over my head. It was then that I could breathe again. I wish I had known about prana back then. I was actually giving up control of my breath and that is why it worked to consciously breathe again.

Think of your breath as your greatest teacher and your greatest resource. You don't need to go searching for some external "silver bullet." We have everything we need with our breath. If you keep prana moving and connect body-mind, a lot of your health issues will get better, you will become smarter, your mental health will improve, and you will be a better lawyer.

Lesson Two Assignment:

These assignments are building on each other. You are still doing the New Billable Hour. You are still practicing your meditation twice daily. And now you are adding a daily pranayama practice. Even if you add just one breath to the end of your meditation session or add one conscious breath to your daily routine, that is sufficient to access your body-mind. Alternately, you can take this breath when you wake up in the morning or before you go to sleep at night. Your body will remember that connection with your breath.

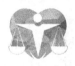

Chapter 6

Lesson Three:
Connect Brain + Gut:
Thinking with your Belly

Hymn to the Belly
Room! room! make room for the bouncing Belly,
First father of sauce and deviser of jelly;
Prime master of arts and the giver of wit,
That found out the excellent engine, the spit,
The plough and the flail, the mill and the hopper,

The hutch and the boulter, the furnace and copper,
The oven, the bavin, the mawkin, the peel,
The hearth and the range, the dog and the wheel.
– Ben Jonson

What is in the belly of the holistic lawyer? In *The New Billable Hour*, I mentioned the "gut-brain" connection. Here, we are continuing to talk about that connection between our brain and our literal gut, including our stomach and digestive system. What do we know? We know that when you are anxious or stressed, your belly suffers. When you are really excited, you have butterflies in your belly. Both of these experiences show up in your belly. Our bellies are important indicators of what is going on in our minds.

We also know about gut feelings. No matter who you are and how heady you are or how much in your brain or intellect you reside, you know what a gut feeling is. You have experienced it in your life. You know what it is to "feel out" a situation. It's not about thinking, it's not about reasoning. It is about you *feeling* it out. You go into a room and feel out what is going on. You can feel other people's energy.

Empathy is another gut feeling where we can *feel* what other people are feeling. Because otherwise, how can we possibly know? We also know when something doesn't "feel right." We feel in our gut, and when it doesn't *feel* right, we know it. We know about how important first impressions are. They stick with us and are usually correct.

We know about love at first sight. People often say "I just knew" when they made an important decision in their lives. They just knew that a person was right for them, or a job was the right job. I knew that my home was right for me when I visited for the first time with my realtor. Whether or not we are correct in the long term, we had some kind of knowing that wasn't intellectual, thinky, or brainy. It was a different kind of thinking. This gut feeling I have described above is not an emotion (which is the next lesson). This is intuition. It is a sense and has been called a "sixth sense." Intuition is basically trusting your gut and letting go.

However, since these intuitive decisions are so fast, they can feel like snap decisions. You get that feeling right away and make that decision right away. But it can be so fast that you don't trust it. We, as lawyers, have been taught (and this idea has been reinforced) that thinking has to be slow and deliberate. We think that making decisions should take time and be calculated. If the decision is made fast, we think it is not a real decision.

As a result, we may overdo it with overthinking. We may overanalyze. We may over-research. We may over-try to find external validation for what we already know. Because we don't trust ourselves, we want someone else to say it, or write about it. We think that slower is superior.

When we reinforce this slow model, we lose the confidence to listen to our own intuition. When we get that gut feeling, we don't trust it. So this lesson is about how to have confidence in your intuition. We don't really know where intuition lives. One idea is that it is in the gut. The research about the gut-brain posits that there is a brain in the gut. So we can say that intuition is in our belly and that is why I call it "thinking with our belly" and getting out of our head. And remember, the ability to have intuition also resides in the right side of the neocortex.

Let me bring this back to the New Billable Hour concept. Since we think slower is superior, the legal system was built on this time model of how long it takes to work on a case. And then we charge by the hour, and that reinforces the measure of taking a long time to do a competent job. And if it doesn't take long to complete a task, you believe you did something wrong. Since you are not meeting your billable hour requirements, you take longer to comply with your assignment. This is going on while your gut is telling you that you already know the answer. We are told not to listen to our gut and that we have to confirm everything. We have to cite things! We have to have references!

One lawyer told me that when she worked for a firm and completed a case, her superiors consistently would tell her there were not enough hours billed. Some law firms have practices of doing unnecessary work or having another lawyer or paralegal redo work to bill more hours. These questionable unethical practices put you, the lawyer, in a difficult position. The client may also question if a lawyer does her job too quickly. Clients may have a notion that lawyers are supposed to take a certain amount of time to do the work. It seems like we have to justify our worth as a lawyer by overdoing it. Lawyer, if you run into these doubts, simply go with your gut. Challenge your externally-imposed doubts and trust your inner wisdom and confidence. And then use that confidence to create innovative ways to both provide high-quality service and also meet the demands of your firm.

When I work with lawyers, I often have them slow their breathing down to their bellies. Then I ask them a question and have them answer from their belly, not their head. I asked one client, who was letting others take advantage of her time and resources at the expense of her law business, what was she afraid of. She relaxed into her belly and declared, "I am afraid of success!" We were both surprised about the honesty and clarity of that declaration. I asked another lawyer why he was avoiding his daily meditation practice. He quieted his mind and spoke his truth from his belly: "I don't want to lose control." The truth was freeing for him and now he is even exploring yoga!

Intuition is following what you already know as opposed to trying to reason your way, which may get you into trouble. You know how your friend sat next to someone on a plane who offered him his dream job? Or when you think about someone and they call or you run into them? That is intuition. Imagine if lawyers like you had the confidence to trust their gut and intuition. What if *you* had that confidence?

Looking at everything as a whole and being mindful and breathing will hone your intuition. This is going to help you decide what to do next. Ultimately, working smarter, not harder is about trusting your gut and intuition to tell you what to do next. Because we waste so much time and get so stressed out because we don't know what to do—we spin out and we don't have a direction. If we can hone this awareness and connection to ourselves, it's a game-changer.

Lesson Three Assignment:

Practice listening to your gut and feeling things out. When you have a gut feeling, stay with it and listen to it before you move on to the next thing. Notice when you have the answer to a problem. Pay attention to how you feel when you enter a courtroom or meet with a client.

To further develop your intuition, remember to integrate both sides of the brain. The right side of the brain is said to be the part where intuition and imagination are born. To activate the right side of your brain, take up a hobby like art, dance, music, or sports. Do things that express your creativity or use both sides of your physical body.

Chapter 7
Lesson Four:
Connect Head + Heart:
Raise Your Emotional IQ

Time Is

Time is
Too Slow for those who Wait,
Too Swift for those who Fear,
Too Long for those who Grieve,
Too Short for those who Rejoice;

But for those who Love,
Time is not.
– Henry van Dyke

I hate it when I waste my time with meaningless drama. The other day I had an interaction with someone and noticed that he was very irritable. So I simply removed myself from the situation and walked away instead of getting wrapped up in his emotions and drama. And I realized right away—"Yay for me!" I thought. I saw clearly that his attitude was about himself and not about me. I did not take the bait! Through awareness we develop compassion for others and for ourselves. Through this emotional intelligence, we can move forward instead of backward or sideways.

I am sure you have already heard of the concept of "emotional intelligence." A big thing for lawyers is that our emotions get in our way and derail and detract from our goal. Then we are not able to be clear-minded and focused to accomplish what we need to do in front of us. And this emotional distraction happens all the time, from judges, opposing counsel, clients, and our own selves. We generate so many emotions against ourselves.

Remember the layers of the brain? When we are emotionally triggered, are we able to move past that part of the brain? It is fun to stay in our emotions because that is where the drama is. It is entertaining, you can find lot of friends to stay there with you, and advertisers are targeting you to stay there. You can watch movies and television all about the drama and stories. You can vent to people and live your life that way.

Alternatively, dear reader, you can take this to the next level and use your emotions as signals. Use them for what they are supposed to be used for. When we have a feeling, it is supposed to just go through us. As we have evolved, this feeling will come in and we notice, "That's interesting" or, "That is a scary thing I should avoid," or, "That is a good thing I should go toward," or, "That is neutral." (You can have neutral feelings, by the way.)

So you have those feelings, and you get motivated to do something, or maybe change the course of what you are doing. It's a signal. However, lawyers like to hold on to our feelings. If the feeling is good, and it goes away, we search out something that will create a feeling that resembles the good feeling we had. We may do this in an unhealthy way. When a bad feeling comes, we either hold onto it or we'll really try to run away from it. However, no matter how much we run, it will keep coming back since we haven't dealt with it.

As discussed in Chapter 2, emotions are temporary and they are meant to move. That is why we are so focused on our breath, because we can breathe through our emotions. They are meant to move. An emotion can be nervousness or anxiety, which can be normalized depending on how you grew up. We think that is how we are supposed to feel all the time, and we don't let those emotions move through. When we were under five years old, we learned a lot about emotions and how to deal with them based on our gender, socioeconomic class, and culture. We learned what our parents, school, and society taught us about emotions and we have these really deep emotional beliefs. The time has come to shift those beliefs.

The next stage of your holistic lawyer evolution is to become aware of your own emotions. Some very intelligent people came up with the concept of emotional intelligence. I like to keep things really simple. The emotional intelligence philosophy has many different emotions you can identify. You can name them all, and analyze them. However, from ancient wisdom, it all comes down to two emotions: love and fear. Love is connectedness to all there is; which is what we want to feel. Fear is disconnected from all there is; and makes us feels alone and separate. Negative feelings are emotions of fear: loneliness, isolation, anger, jealousy, and hate. Positive feelings are emotions of love: joy, gratitude, care, and generosity.

Of course there are so many emotions in the middle, so please allow yourself to feel them all. Since you are a lawyer, resist the urge to analyze every emotion that comes through. Just identify it and let it go through. We are using our higher brain, the one used for wisdom and higher order thinking, to observe our emotions as they come up. We become observers so that we are not pulled into the drama. We've all been in the drama and it's addictive. It's very stimulating, interesting, and also exhausting. So then we create drama around being exhausted. Drama is all the stories that we have created to entertain ourselves and avoid leveling up.

What if you pulled back from the drama? If you can find this place, you will bring people to your level of calmness. You can truly influence those around you. When I meet with lawyers who are stressed out and imbalanced, that is when I have the opportunity to truly maintain my center. It is my responsibility to stay calm because if I allow myself to get pulled into the drama, I am not serving. Imagine the impact you could have on *your* clients if *you* came from a place of calm.

When you find your authentic self, you can bring the room down to that place of equanimity and stability. This is how, as a true lawyer and leader, you are going to change the planet. If you can do that in the courtroom, in your client communication, with opposing counsel when they are yelling at you, you will change the world. You may have seen luminaries like the Dalai Lama, Mahatma Gandhi, and Thich Nhat Hanh interact with others—they are so stable and even-keeled. This is powerful beyond measure. We get caught up as lawyers thinking that we are supposed to be angry and fighting all the time. Yes, our role is often as fighter and advocate. But it's a choice when you need to fight. By choosing your battles, you are less affected by other people or external factors.

So how do we get there? We start with the meditation and mindfulness that we have been doing. Then, over time, you notice your emotions and let them move through you. If you have been doing sitting meditation, a lot of emotions are coming and going. That is why my preference for you is sitting meditation. Take some time each day to stop moving and doing and just sit with yourself. By sitting, we can watch our emotions. Since we are sitting and not moving, we can let the emotions move. Over time, you will lose the desire to hold on to the emotions. After a while you will simply observe your anger and sadness as it comes through you.

Lesson Four Assignment:

Identify and note down at least one emotion you feel every day. You can either get very specific or break it down to love and fear. Practice noticing your emotions and observing them from a different angle. Remember to breathe while you are identifying and noting.

Chapter 8
Lesson Five:
Depose Yourself:
The Self-Inquiry Process

Ultimately
He tried to spit out the truth;
Dry mouthed at first,
He drooled and slobbed in the end;
Truth dribbling his chin.

– Ernest Hemingway

Telling ourselves the truth is really hard. Even though we seek out truth for a living, seeing our own truth is another animal. We each have unique story, and every single event, circumstance, coincidence, failure, insight, trauma, and success brought you here to this exact moment. Yes, the exact moment you are reading this. Because that is all there is. This moment. Remember that everything, all the causes and conditions, brought us to this moment. And when you forget, take a breath, meditate, and recalibrate your perspective.

As you progress on your path, you will be a guide to others who are behind you, and to those who are behind them. That's our purpose, to keep moving forward because there are people behind us who we are guiding, whether we know it or not. Even though this sounds so simple, we have sticky parts. I like to call these "pain cycles" These are cycles that keep repeating themselves; we keep making the same mistakes, hurting ourselves and people around us, repeatedly. These pain cycles can lead to physical illness, mental illness, addiction—all merely symptoms of pain cycles that we have not addressed.

And there is a lot of money being made to treat these symptoms. Can't find love? Use a dating service! Not making enough money? Hire a business coach! Not making it to the gym? Just get a personal trainer! All of these services are great and I have bought them myself for tremendous benefit. However, if we are aligned and have cleaned out our past, those obstacles get a lot easier to overcome, and solutions come more naturally. We don't need to be "coached" or have someone tell us what to do. Also, if you resolve one symptom without addressing the cause, it's like the game "whack-a-mole"—it will pop up somewhere else in your life. Your pain cycle will show up in another part of your life.

You are so brave to have gotten this far. You chose to take a deep look at yourself, unfiltered, and you have been observing your breath, thoughts, and emotions. This is not easy, especially for lawyers. I hope you noticed that the emotions and the thoughts that go with them are temporary and fleeting. We only have this moment. Thoughts are about the past or the future. So, all we have is this moment in the present and if we are really present, everything moves all the time, because the present keeps moving. It's not a fixed place.

Also, you probably notice some emotions that are stuck. The emotions can be moving, but some just are really sticky. Remember the pain cycles? That is why they are stuck. Pain cycles make us go into the past and future.

The good news is that whatever you have been through, it has brought you to becoming a successful lawyer! And that's why you are here. You can complain all you want, but really you are doing well.

We learned how to cope with difficulty by going into our heads, being really smart and good students. We learned how to get external validation. We learned how to make walls around our hearts! I am joking, but this how we lawyers got the reputation that we take emotion out of situations. And we kind of need to, to do the work we do—no matter what kind of law you are practicing. I just want to celebrate that, right? It is a skill that we learned to be successful to help ourselves and help each other.

However, as discussed in the last chapter, our emotional IQ is not that great because we have stuffed that part of us away. It's time to up-level. The way to really up-level is to take a deep look at ourselves, to depose ourselves and clean out this emotional backlog. The pain cycles have a lot of emotions that we haven't dealt with. The emotions go way back, and they are no one's fault. The way to clean out this backlog is to ask ourselves questions on an emotional level.

Let's peel back the layers. When you are feeling an emotion, think about these four questions:

1. What do I really feel?
2. What do I need?
3. Why am I holding on to this feeling?
4. What would happen if I let it go?

This is the Self-Inquiry Process. It is healing. You can reintegrate part of you that has been wounded and separated from you—and use that insight to help others. What gets really great is that when you process your emotions, you begin to develop compassion for others. You will notice that when others express negative emotions, there must be something beneath that. And that is how we are going to heal ourselves and others.

Those stuck emotions are great information. The Self-Inquiry Process is about getting to the root of what is causing all of our physical problems, mental health problems, and addictions. So these problems are just signals for which emotions and situations stick with us. The trigger could be that your client didn't even thank you for the good job you did. And you feel that resentment all day. It could be that the judge did not grant your case. All day you grumble, "The judge is unfair!" It could be that opposing counsel is not competent. My feeling about others' incompetence is something that can still set me off. "I have worked so hard to be competent, why aren't others doing the same?"—is a common thought of mine.

For an example of how the Self-Inquiry Process works, let's take the one where your client did not thank you for a job well done. Believe me, I have felt this numerous times. Let's go:

1. What do I really feel? Initially I think I am angry or pissed off. But under that I may feel hurt, betrayed, unappreciated, or just something as simple as lonely.

2. What do I need? I need validation, appreciation, connection, and love. We have all the tools, we don't need anyone to give that to us. However, I can also inquire whether I can give myself what I need or ask for that need to be met by someone I trust. Being very independent myself, I forget that seeking out the help of others is paramount in the healing process. Either directly or indirectly, you can ask for your need as opposed to letting that sticky emotion stay with you.

3. Why am I holding on to this feeling? It is usually an old hurt story, that I have not felt appreciated or not

felt loved or connected. Then I keep hitting against this story. Instead of resolving that need by finding a healthy way to get that need met or giving it to ourselves, we are doing the same pain cycle—which not only causes pain to ourselves, but to everyone around us. When we are angry, we react in ways that hurt other people, like the client who didn't do anything wrong.

4. What would happen if I let this feeling go? I would feel out of control, I would feel weak, I would feel like I lost my edge, I would feel afraid of the unknown, I have been doing this for so long! It's so comfortable to react in this old way. And if I let it go, I will be able to create space for something new.

This exercise will get easier with practice. I'm not suggesting you do it daily. But try it regularly. When you feel a sticky emotion, use this process to, well, process it! Instead of trying to escape it, pacify the feelings, vent it out (which doesn't really work), project on to someone else, or numb yourself with alcohol, food, drugs, shopping, or television, how about going deeper within? This is not for the timid. And you won't do it every time. You will still want some escape sometimes. This takes a lot of strength. And I know you are very strong.

As you continue to practice this, it will get easier. Remember to incorporate all your lessons: the New Billable Hour, your daily mindfulness, your breathing, listening to your intuition, and using your emotional intelligence. You have to be in touch with yourself, otherwise it is not going to work. Let's become friends with ourselves and go deeper into who we really are.

Lesson Five Assignment:

Begin a journaling practice using the Self-Inquiry Process for when your emotions get sticky. You are still doing all the other lessons. You are still identifying your emotions. You are still observing them. But let's see which ones stick. There are so many present moments throughout the day and so many opportunities to observe. Most of what we feel is neutral. You may think, "Oh that happened" or, "I saw that" or, "That upset me, but I recovered" or, "I was so excited about this, and the feeling went away." The emotions are moving through during the day. At the end of the day, however, some of the emotions stick. When that happens, use the Self-Inquiry Process.

NOTE: I know that journaling can be triggering for lawyers. You may be afraid someone will find the evidence of your innermost feelings. All I can say is to trust that your truth, if meant for healing, will be used for just that. If you don't feel comfortable writing this exercise, you can record your voice speaking the answers. You can also write it down and destroy the evidence. Or you can type it on your computer, phone, or tablet and then delete.

Chapter 9
Lesson Six:
Find Your Purpose:
Your Mission Statement

The Road Not Taken
I shall be telling this with a sigh
Somewhere ages and ages hence:
Two roads diverged in a wood, and I,
I took the one less traveled by,
And that has made all the difference.
– Robert Frost

At every fork in the road of your life, you have a choice. And the lifelong lessons of this program give you the tools to make the best choice possible for you on *your* path. As you know, the lessons of this program build on each other. Moreover, the lessons are also interwoven. They are happening simultaneously. So when you are thinking about your emotions, you are breathing. When you are figuring out how to depose yourself, you are going with your gut feeling. All of these lessons are interwoven.

For many personal growth programs, usually the steps start with your mission statement or a vision to set your intention. For you, lawyer, we started with broad concepts and then gotten down into the granular. This is because for the lawyers I have worked with, this idea of a mission statement and vision planning is strange and foreign. We have been on this career track where we have been told what to do by others, and we have told *ourselves* what to do. And as I discussed earlier, our creativity has been diluted. Now that you have learned how to access your whole brain and self, it's time to find your purpose by creating your mission statement.

Mission statements are not new. It is common for businesses and professionals to spend time creating a strategic plan or setting goals in the long or short term. However, for lawyers, this tool is not part of our rubric. We let a lot of external circumstances dictate what we do. The reason to have a mission is to give you internal direction for where you are headed and to remind you of your goals when you get distracted. You must know where you are going.

There are so many opportunities for distraction to pull you away from where you are going. But the life that you want to live, where you enjoy yourself, have loving relationships, and make a difference in the world—is completely possible, if you can stay focused. All the ills of the world are caused by distraction. You may be distracted by what you think you should be doing, what other people are doing, and other people's ideas of success.

Further, without your own vision or mission, you are going to be easily swayed by opposing counsel, judges, clients, the ever-changing law, the media, and what other people think about you. You are constantly going to be pulled in all these directions because you don't have a focus to stay grounded. I know that for so long your focus has been on becoming a lawyer. And you did it! You are a successful lawyer! This identity as a lawyer has given you purpose.

Despite having this identity and purpose as a lawyer, there is still so much discontent in the legal profession. In our current times, it's no longer enough to just say, "I am a lawyer." A lawyer is one role you play for some *higher* purpose or mission. And if you don't know what that purpose is, life can be very unsatisfying and stressful. It can feel like a letdown because you worked so hard to become a lawyer. You had to jump through so many hoops to get here. It's no small thing. Your mission statement thus far has been to be a lawyer. And now that you have been practicing law for a while, it's time to up-level as you move forward in the profession and in your personal life.

Everyone has an agenda. And if you don't have your own, you will be pulled into other people's agendas. You do need to have your own—it's not selfish. The mindfulness techniques that you have been incorporating into your life are meant to give you the confidence to find that knowing of *your* agenda, of *your* vision, of *your* mission.

Your mission statement is for your whole life, not just for being a lawyer. Once you have your mission statement, you can practice law in a way where being a lawyer is your vehicle to get there. Of course, there are other vehicles too, and you will bring your whole being into everything you do when you know your mission.

The good news is that you already know your purpose! You have just forgotten. It is also common to cover up that knowing with fears, anxiety, expectations, and external stress. So you may need to go deep inside to find your purpose. This process is fun, and it doesn't hurt at all.

This exercise is not a one-time thing. You'll do it many times in your life. Some people do it every calendar year. Others line it up with their quarterly business planning. Whatever works for you should involve revisiting the process as you learn and grow. Your purpose may stay the same, but how you are going to get there may change. Often people do it backward. They think, "I am in the wrong job!" or, "I don't know if I want to be a lawyer," or, "Something is wrong in my personal life, my relationships aren't working out." These are symptoms of whether you are really on track toward *your* vision and your purpose— moment to moment, breath by breath. You cannot do this visioning practice if you are not mindful. So if you have not even tried to integrate the other lessons in your life, this is going to be difficult. Your results will come from your old programming and not from your deep sense of self.

If you can let go, the process will be very natural. I do this process regularly with my lawyer clients and what they come up with constantly blows my mind. They are able to peel away the layers to get to why they are here and how they will bring that purpose to their law practice. I see the lawyers struggle by "thinking" of their purpose using only part of their brain. Then, I ask them to close their eyes, put their hands on their belly, and take a few deep breaths. And then their mission statement easily comes to them.

When you have identified your purpose, your life as a lawyer will improve. Your interactions with your clients, your co-workers, judges, and clerks will have more meaning. You will enter every situation with confidence. By being present in your role as lawyer, you will feel happy and satisfied.

But if you are not being mindful about how you practice law, and you're just living these stories and distracted, then there will be a lot of discontent. Whatever you decide to do in your life, whether you decide to leave the law, stay in the law, change where you are, or just change your attitude—you are a lawyer. You chose to become a lawyer.

You went through all the steps to become a lawyer—for a reason.

And now is the time to remember that reason. Our profession has forgotten. That is why I am reaching out to you, lawyer, and why I work with lawyers. Something deep inside you called for you to use your privilege and your unique skills to serve. When you are mindful in every moment, you will get to your core of who you really are. The essence of being a holistic lawyer is being mindful from moment to moment. If you can cultivate mindfulness in your life more and more—you will have clarity, ease, and success. Whatever you truly want will manifest.

Lesson Six Assignment:

Create your own personal mission statement from a place of mindfulness. After a session of meditation or merely taking a few breaths to be present in the moment, ask yourself, "What is my purpose?" Simply experience what comes to you. This is a practice in letting go and trusting the answer will come. Boil it down to a few words or a short sentence.

Then create a reminder of your vision statement. This can be anything from a sticky note (physical or virtual) to a keepsake token reminder. This will be something that you look at every day to remind you of your vision and that *every* choice you make, everything that you do, will be guided by your own personal mission statement.

Chapter 10
The Future of Competence & Ethics

On Freedom
*And what is it but fragments of your own self you
would discard that you may become free?
If it is an unjust law you would abolish, that law was
written with your own hand upon your own forehead.
You cannot erase it by burning your law books
nor by washing the foreheads of your judges,
though you pour the sea upon them.*
– Kahlil Gibran

Lawyer, you have willingly accepted the lifestyle and philosophy of overworking. It has actually been *your* choice, over and over, to practice law that way. You have followed the example of lawyers before you for how to establish your competence and to be ethical by overworking. And this overworking has painted you in a corner of sorts. I like to think of it as a self-imposed prison, which is not locked. I see time and time again lawyers choosing to live this life of stress and overwhelm. And that way of life is certainly an option—it has served you well until now.

I also have the honor to guide lawyers to discover a new way to be a lawyer. This new way involves letting go and trusting that working *harder* is not the way to lawyer freedom. The future of being a competent and ethical lawyer involves using your whole brain and self to work *smarter*. The future is the holistic lawyer. Becoming a holistic lawyer can seem like a huge responsibility, because it is. You have infinite power to create your own destiny, but you must choose to do so. We make this choice over and over, moment by moment.

Operating on a limited brain can mean that fear, worry, and perfectionism paralyze you. As you know, using the programs in this book and my previous book arm you with the tools necessary to see clearly and eliminate these limitations. Instead of focusing on the outcome, you change how you use your brain and self in every moment. By taking yourself off of autopilot so you can fly to freedom, the possibilities of your life open up.

I know that change is daunting, but as you chisel away at old thought patterns and behaviors, you will create a flow that will allow more flow. It's like when you de-gunk the pipes, everything flows better and continues to do so. You are paving the way for the path ahead. And it takes guts.

If you have the guts to think with your belly and connect with yourself in a meaningful way, you will be a holistic lawyer who will greatly impact the world—by actually working less. Working smarter, not harder is just that. What if we could get bigger impact by doing less? Doing less does not mean you are lazy or incompetent or unethical.

In this final chapter, I would like to directly address ethics and competence. Your state licensing authority probably has continuing legal education requirements on these topics. As lawyers, we are each required to follow the professional rules in order to zealously advocate for our clients.

Rule 1.1 of the American Bar Association's Model Rules of Professional Conduct defines competence:

> *A lawyer shall provide competent representation to a client. Competent representation requires the legal knowledge, skill, thoroughness and preparation reasonably necessary for the representation.*

The rest of the Model Rules describe how to ethically do this.

Unfortunately, as I have explained in this book, we have interpreted these rules to mean we must overwork. As a result we have been only using parts of our brains and selves. The soft skills addressed in this book have been dismissed as "nice to have" but not as *required* for competence.

Well, holistic lawyer, what if you could be *more* competent and ethical by working *less* hard? By integrating the lessons of the Holistic Lawyer Program, you will be more efficient by using your whole brain. Not only will you be more efficient in your tasks and more productive on your cases, you will see things you did not see before. You will more easily see both liabilities and solutions to problems. You will be able to access more of your own knowledge and confidence. You will be more skilled in your craft. And yes, you will have the acumen to be more focused which will make you more thorough and hence, more prepared and competent.

I know that this new way of thinking and practicing law may cause you to meet certain challenges from others in the field. I can imagine that your supervisors and colleagues may think you are shirking your responsibilities with your efficient and good nature. Taking time for yourself may be met with disdain and jealousy. You may lose the praise you have received for overworking to the point of exhaustion. You may regret giving up distractions and become anxious with your newfound productivity and ease in your work.

Or, dear lawyer, you may choose to go back to your old comfortable ways in your corner prison.

I understand. And that is why I ask you to come back to this book when such backslides happen. Remember what you learned to allow you to enjoy practicing law. At these times, you can restart the entire program or go back to a lesson that you specifically need when circumstances get especially stressful in your life. And always go back to basics. Take a few minutes or a few breaths to come back to the present moment so you can respond to what is happening right now instead of reacting with old patterns.

This process to a new way of lawyering, of being a holistic lawyer, requires that you really want it. And if you don't, that is fine too. But if you hear that little voice inside telling you that it's time for a new paradigm for how you practice law—listen to it. Find a community of like-minded lawyers. Work with teachers and mentors to keep you on track. You are not alone and it is time for you to step up and into the next version of you. The world is waiting.

Conclusion

Human Being
The felt body holds
the vagus nerve
from stem to stern,
the two legs dangling down.
Above, between the ears,
street-smarts galore.
Below, the heart and belly,
loving, deep and wise.
– Angie Boissevain

Y ou may have noticed that I dedicated this book to my longtime Zen teacher and poet, Angie Boissevain. I shared with her how I wanted to start each chapter with a poem so you, the reader, could access more of your brain through the magic of poetry. I asked if she had written any poems about the brain—and wouldn't you know, she wrote the above original poem for this book and for you. And since it just sums it all up, I put it with my Conclusion.

In my first book, I described how I began my own journey into meditation and mindfulness. It started with curiosity, then learning the tools, and then finding teachers and community. In this life journey, everything we learn and everyone we encounter becomes part of the whole human beings we truly are. As you move forward on your path, dear reader, you will begin to notice there are others behind you on your path. You can call them followers or see them as teachers. For me, my readers and clients are my inspiration to find new ways to teach and learn.

Thank you for reading this book and learning about the holistic lawyer program. As I explained at the beginning, now that you have read the book through once, go back and take some time with each lesson. While the lessons build on each other, you can always go back and relearn the lessons that call to you. There may be something that is more interesting and something you may need to be with for a long time before you can move on to the next step. You can now go backward and forward.

I wish you well as a holistic lawyer moving forward to use your whole brain and self to work smarter, not harder. I wish you a life of balance and ease. Please go forth and be an example to other lawyers, and to your clients who are suffering and going through a lot of conflict. Let's change the legal profession and how we view ourselves as lawyers, and how others view us. Let's get out of this self-imposed prison of overworking. Let's make the legal profession more desirable and fulfilling. Let's accept our role as leaders and make our lawyer legacy something to be proud of.

Further Reading

Buddha's Brain by Rick Hanson
Super Brain by Deepak Chopra

Acknowledgements

This book would not be possible without the Author Incubator team. Thank you Angela Lauria, Ora North, Bethany Davis, and everyone else who touched my book and mission.

Thank you Dr. Ron Stotts for pushing me to new levels and for teaching me how to be gentle in the process.

To the lawyers who trusted me and signed up for the first holistic lawyer program before I had created it: Eliana Maruri, Jason Redula, Jeraline Singh Edwards, and Victoria Slater Giambra. You all graduated from the New Billable Hour program and wanted more and so I created this book and program. Thank you for your openness, curiosity, and confidence to go deeper into yourself as a lawyer. You are paving the way for many others to follow.

To the Morgan James Publishing team: Special thanks to David Hancock, CEO & Founder for believing in me and my message. To my Author Relations Manager, Margo Toulouse, thanks for making the process seamless and easy. Many more thanks to everyone else, but especially Jim Howard, Bethany Marshall, and Nickcole Watkins.

And my sincere appreciation for all the lawyers out there who are brave enough to seek a new way to work and live. I applaud you and this book is for you.

Thank You!

You are well on your way to becoming a holistic lawyer and using your whole brain and self to work smarter, not harder.

To help you work on the lessons in this book, you can download a free printable workbook at www.theholistic lawyer.com.

If you want to continue the conversation, you can also email me directly at ritu@theholisticlawyer.com.

Wishing you a productive and rewarding legal career,
Ritu Goswamy, Esq.

About the Author

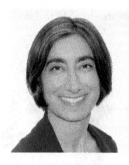

Ritu Goswamy, Esq., is a lawyer and productivity consultant for lawyers. She teaches lawyers the tools to work smarter and be more productive for work-life balance. Ritu is the creator of the New Billable Hour program (level one), which helps lawyers increase their productivity by billing themselves first. She teaches this system directly to lawyers in a way that is engaging, fun, and practical. By prioritizing our needs in an efficient way, we are able to then respond to other demands on our time. Due to the success of the New Billable Hour program, Ritu created the level two holistic lawyer program where lawyers can go deeper into how to work less and have a bigger impact in their professional and personal lives. Ritu's philosophy is to shift from the reactive training we have as lawyers to live more intentionally the life we desire.

Ritu holds a bachelor of arts in psychology from Barnard College and a juris doctorate and master of social work from Boston College. She is a Registered Yoga Teacher with Yoga Alliance and a certified Ayurvedic Health Counselor. Ritu lives amongst the coastal redwoods in the Santa Cruz Mountains, CA.

Website: www.theholisticlawyer.com

Email: ritu@theholisticlawyer.com

LinkedIn: http://www.linkedin.com/in/ritu-goswamy/

Facebook: www.facebook.com/ritugo

Instagram: @ritugoswamy

CPSIA information can be obtained
at www.ICGtesting.com
Printed in the USA
JSHW021830010323
38371JS00004B/508